The

Fit

Traveler

Take Your Workout With You

by fitness globetrotters
Kari Eide & Lissa Mueller

ISBN: 1-929170-17-3

Library of Congress Congress Control 2005909807

Art direction and photography: Robert Brekke
Cover design: Chuck Donald

IMPORTANT INFORMATION:
While this book provides you with guidance and inspiration in traveling and staying fit, it is not meant as a substitute for expert medical attention or advice. Always consult with your physician before undertaking any exercise or dietary program. The stretch bands included with this book are made of **Latex** which has been known to cause allergic reactions in some people. Keep bands properly stored and out of reach from **children** to avoid accidental suffocation or strangulation. Always inspect bands for wear and tear before commencing a workout—replace old, damaged, or worn-out bands.

Presented by The Fitness Boutique, LLC.

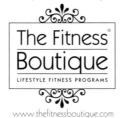

The Fitness® Boutique
LIFESTYLE FITNESS PROGRAMS

www.thefitnessboutique.com

PUBLISHERS DESIGN GROUP
Roseville, California
1.800.587.6666
www.publishersdesign.com

Printed in China

The Fit Traveler

Take Your Workout With You

there's hope

Your prayers have been answered. This is your guide for traveling and staying fit. You will really enjoy this guide. Think of it as the little workout book that can go anywhere—and it really, truly works! I use it, love it, and get huge benefits from it.

Here is my story about hope, and finding a way to workout no matter what the situation might be. I have been an exercise junkie most of my life. I love to run, lift weights and take aerobics classes. Recently though, I was in a car accident and all of these activities came to a screeching halt—no pun intended.

The accident caused severe injuries to my right foot, heel, and ankle, and I had to undergo reconstructive surgery. I spent a lot of time in bed and was devastated by my inability to exercise.

My girlfriend Lissa, who owns the local gym, came to visit me and tried to lift my spirits. She brought me an exercise band. Lissa thought that some training with the band while I was bed ridden would give me the mental as well as physical therapy I needed. The band was a great way for me to maintain my upper body strength since I was not able to do any of my regular fitness routines.

I used the band every day and was able to identify several exercises that worked my biceps, triceps, shoulders and back. By varying where I held the ends of the band, I could increase or decrease the amount of resistance and ended up seeing amazing results. The muscles in my upper body became much more toned and defined. It was also easy for me to do this while lying down in bed or sitting in a chair in my family room. This made it very easy for me to continue my workouts.

Nine months after the car accident my family and I took a vacation. Since I had just begun to exercise again I was worried about traveling and not being able to workout. When I pack for traveling I do not usually pack gym equipment, running shoes and exercise clothes. There is never enough room for all of it and, often the hotels we stay at lack a workout facility anyway.

This time, things were different. I made the decision to pack my band and found it to be the perfect workout equipment to use while I was on the road. Not only did it take up a tiny amount of space, but it allowed me to work out without ever leaving the hotel room. During that vacation, (and several others), I would often work out while my kids were resting, or any other time I had a few free minutes.

In this guide, Lissa and I put together all of the upper body strength training exercises I did during my rehabilitation, as well as the exercises I do while I am on the road. By doing these you will be able to maintain and gain muscle strength in your lower and upper body. We have included a great abdominal section as well. We also thought it would be a great idea to include helpful hints for dieting while you're on the road.

For those times you are not traveling and would just like to start exercising at home, this system works well too. You can do your strength training without a huge investment in free weights or having to leave your home to hit the gym.

To your health and happiness,

Kari

ready,

set.....

workout

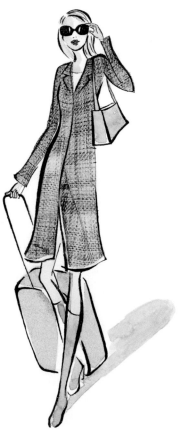

GETTING STARTED

Before beginning your workout, make sure that you have checked with your doctor and have approval to begin a physical regimen.

PROPER POSTURE

- Nice tall and straight posture, bring shoulders back and down.
- Stand in front of a mirror to check for proper body and wrist positioning.
- Make sure you move in a slow and controlled manner.
- Keep neck and face relaxed.
- Hold in your stomach muscles without limiting your breath or raising your shoulders.

THE PLAN

While away from home (entire routine takes approximately 30 minutes):
  (Program should include 3-minute warm-up and 2-minute cool-down sessions.)
  • Complete one set of 15 repetitions of every exercise.
  • Have enough tension on the band to fatigue before 20 repetitions.
  • To add resistance as you get stronger, wrap the band around your hand so
    that you increase the tension in the band. You can also hold the band fur-
    ther down to make the exercise more challenging. Increasing the tension in
    the band works the same as stepping up in the amount of weights you
    would be using if you were using traditional dumbbells.

While at home (you can vary the routine time from 30 to 45 minutes):
  If you would like to incorporate this fitness program into your daily life at
  home, begin with 15 minutes of cardiovascular activity such as a brisk
  walk, bike ride, or jogging in place. During your first workout session you
  should complete three sets of 15 repetitions for each upper body exercise.
  During your next workout, complete your cardio activity and then do the
  lower body exercises. Alternating the targeted muscle groups in this way
  lets those muscles worked during your previous session rest and rebuild.
  You can follow either the upper or lower body strength training with the
  abdominal section workout (see sample home routine below).

SAMPLE HOME ROUTINE

SUN	MON	TUE	WED	THU	FRI	SAT
15 MIN CARDIO	15 MIN CARDIO	15 MIN CARDIO	REST	15 MIN CARDIO	15 MIN CARDIO	15 MIN CARDIO
UPPER BODY	LOWER BODY	UPPER BODY		LOWER BODY	UPPER BODY	LOWER BODY
	ABS			ABS		ABS

upper
body

In the following chapter you will be working your biceps, triceps, shoulders, and back. Please remember, this isn't a race. Use slow and controlled movements and really focus on the muscle group you are working. What helped me was visualizing how I would have been doing this same exercise if I were using a machine or free weights. This technique can help you maintain the proper form and work the targeted muscle area safely and efficiently. (When possible, the best way to do any of the exercises is to position yourself in front of a mirror.)

CHEST

PECTORAL "FLYS"

With band secured by door hinge, leg of bed or a bar, grip band with elbow slightly bent or "soft elbow," palms facing each other (1a). Arms should be open wide, chest height. Press together towards midline of your body as if you are wrapping your arms around a beach ball (1b).

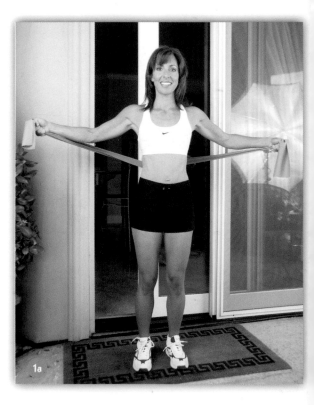

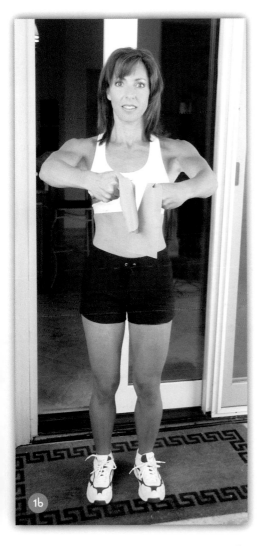

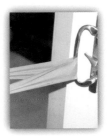

Example of how to secure band.

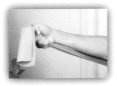

Make sure wrists are straight

9

PUSH UPS

Using a chair or the floor, place hands shoulder width apart, arms straight, elbows unlocked. Place knees on the floor, or if you can, come up on your toes (2a). Bend your arms, keeping head aligned with the spine, and your abdominals held in. Your chest should almost be touching the chair when you are in the down position. (2b). Come back up to starting position and repeat for 15 reps or until muscles are fatigued.

Ensure body is completely aligned in a "plank" position. Make sure gluteus doesn't come up and that most of weight is not on your feet.

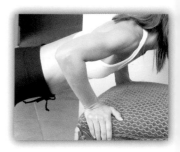

Make sure elbows point backwards, not out to the sides.

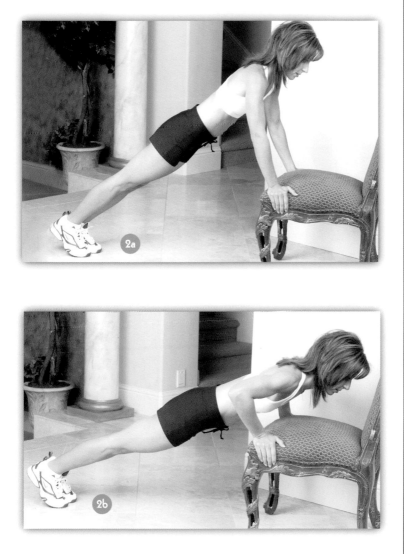

SHOULDERS

LATERAL RAISES

Grip bandwhile standing on it with feet shoulder width apart, lift hands away from the sides of the body, to approximately shoulder height (3a). Elbows should remain slightly bent. Raise hands out and away from the body (3b). Lower arms down to starting position. Do not allow the hands to rest on the outer thigh in the down position.

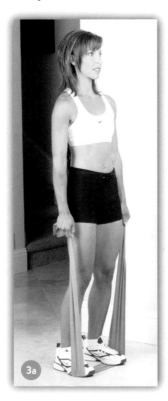

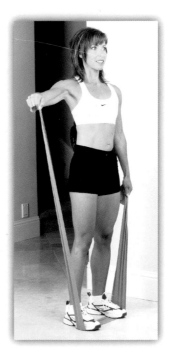

Vary exercises by doing all right side reps, then all left side reps

UpperBody

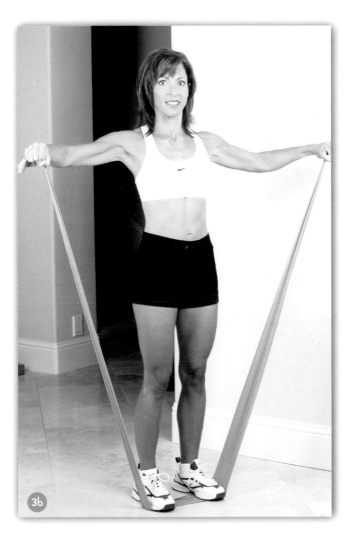

ANTERIOR RAISES

Grip band while standing on the middle of it with feet shoulder width apart, palms facing the front of upper leg (4a). Lift hands shoulder height (4b). Do not allow hands to rest on legs between repetitions. Either alternate right/left or lift simultaneously.

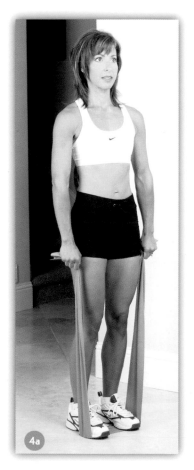

4a

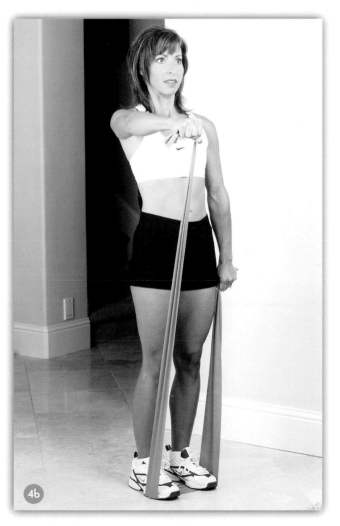

BACK

VERTICAL ROW

Secure band to door handle or hinge. Grip band, step back arm's length away and plant feet as shown (5a). Pull hands toward body, pressing the chest slightly forward without arching the lower back (5b). Allow the elbows to run back past the ribs, "squeezing" the shoulder blades in towards the spine. Slowly return to the starting position.

Other ways to
secure your band

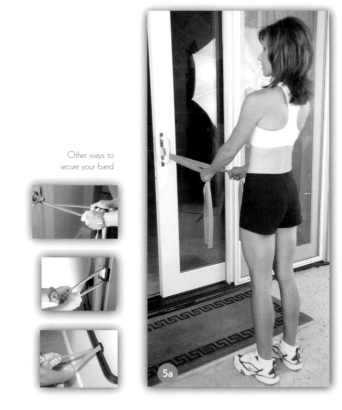

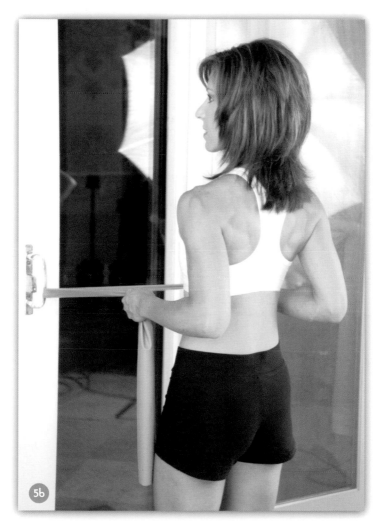

UPRIGHT ROW

Stand on band with feet hip width apart, without "locking" the knees (6a). With palms facing the front of your body, raise the elbows as far as possible without "shrugging" the shoulders (6b). Keep your neck long (ears away from shoulders). Hands close to the front of the body, wrists in alignment with forearm.

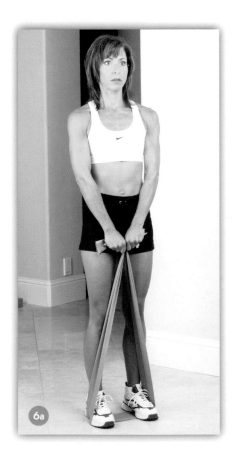

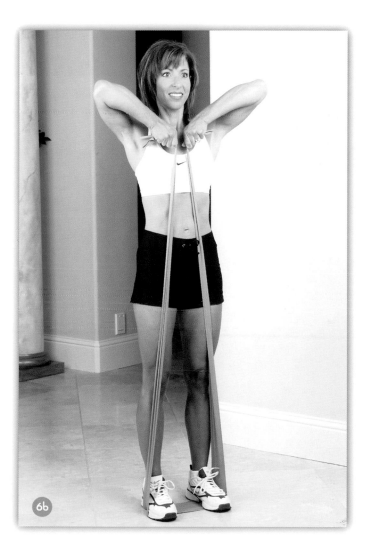

BICEPS

BICEP CURLS

Grip ends of band, place under one shoe and move the other foot back as shown. Space hands shoulder width apart with palms forward and rotated away from body without arching the back (7a). Then pull the hands up, just outside the shoulder, bending at the elbows (7b). Straighten the arms, keep the wrists from flexing (bending).

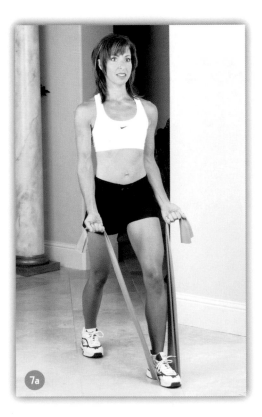

7a

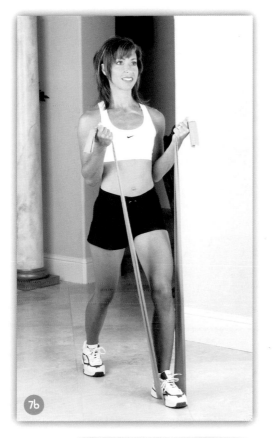

7b

Notice straight arm and
wrist tension.

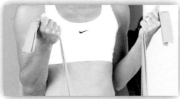

HAMMER CURLS

Grip band with hands shoulder width apart, palms facing inward. Place band under shoes (8a). Rotate palm toward shoulder, bend elbow. Lower one arm, bending at the elbow to the thigh and back up again (8b). Repeat with other arm.

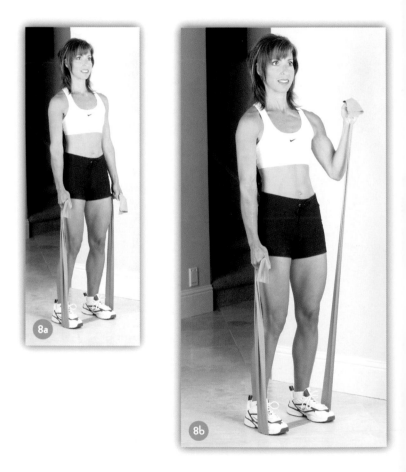

TRICEPS

KICKBACKS

Grip band in both hands holding on hand by your ear, and the other hand behind your back on the opposite side of the body. Hand by head moves over head by extending the elbow (9a). Use full range of motion, offering resistance from your behind the back grip of the band. Return to 90° flexion at the elbow and press into full extension (9b). Repeat. Change grip and perform described exercise on the other side.

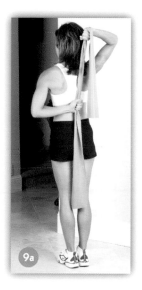

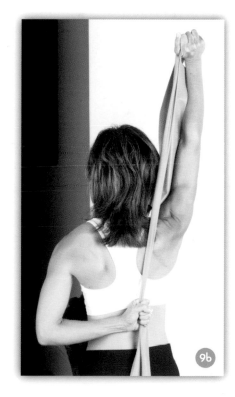

DIPS

Place heels of hands on top of step, stair, or chair (make sure it will support your weight). Bending elbow back, close to the body "chicken wing" (10a). Control descent to 90° angle at joint and press elbow into extension (10b). Fully focus on the back of your arms. You should feel your bodyweight shift "up and down" not "forward and back."

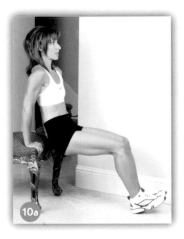

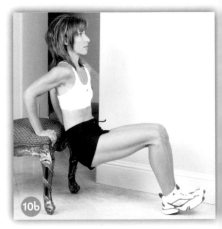

Notice that back is erect and away from the chair. Elbows are straight back.

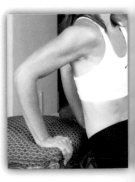

lower
body

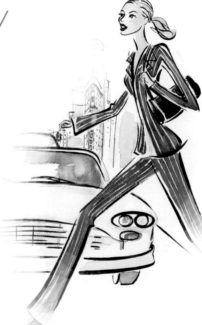

Yes this works. The following lower-body routine is one I do at home as well as when I am traveling. I don't use any lower body workout machines. I follow these exercises four times per week and am very happy with the results. As with the previous section, you also want to make sure to "pause and squeeze" the muscle group you are working. This means slow down each movement and tighten up the muscle you are focusing on.

You'll be working your entire lower body. While doing these moves do not allow your knees to go past your toes when bending. This puts undo strain on your knees and also prohibits you from achieving proper weight distribution on the proper areas.

Add resistance as you progress. The lower body has always been a tricky area for me, I blame it on heredity—okay—and diet.

QUADRICEPS (front of leg)

LUNGES

Place band under front foot. Grip band creating resistance and move into proper lunge position (1a). The front knee should not extend over the toe and the back knee should create a 90° angle of flexion (1b). Keep the sense of uprightness with the upper body (1c). Repeat with the other leg in front. (If needed, bent arms may be raised to shoulder level to increase stability.)

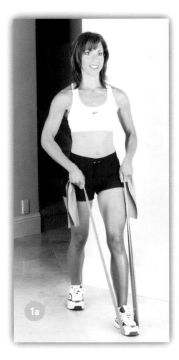

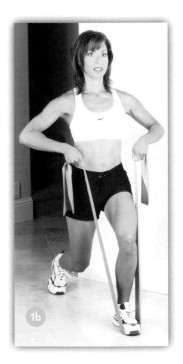

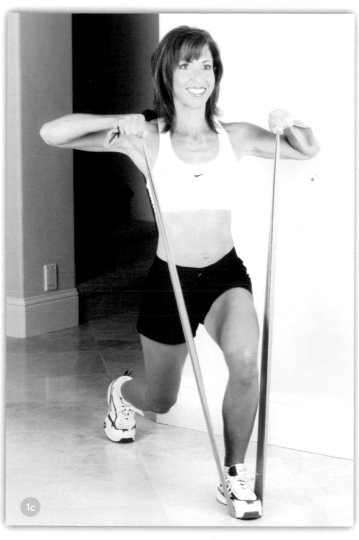

STANDING LEG RAISES

Step one foot forward onto middle of band, holding ends in both hands (2a). Lift and lower this leg, keeping it straight and holding the band tightly. (2b). This exercise has an added benefit of increasing the strength of the supporting leg and improving your balance. Repeat with other leg.

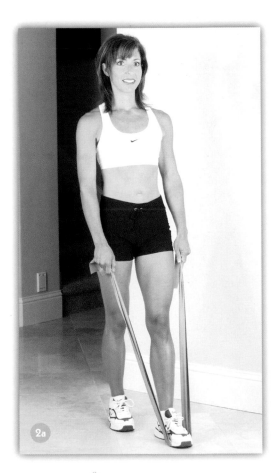

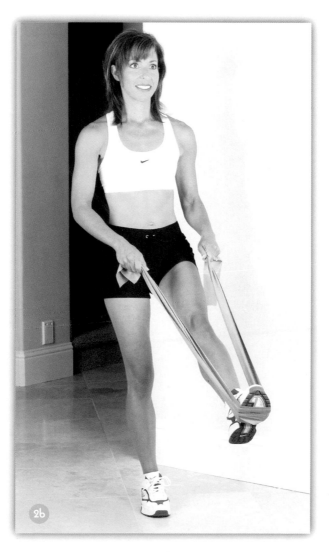

HAMSTRINGS (Back of leg)

STANDING LEG CURLS

Attach band to ankle to create a leash-like device (3a). Grip other end of band and stand on the band to create tension (3b). Place "leashed" ankle behind body, lead with the heel toward the buttock by bending the knee. Return to starting position. Repeat with other leg.

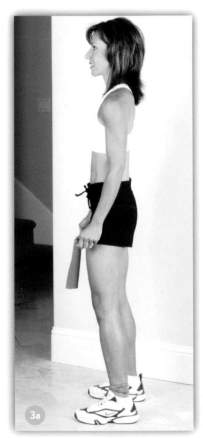

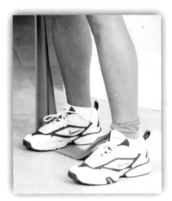

Detail of attached band.
If you wrap the band loosely around the ankle and then tie a double knot, you will avoid cutting off circulation.

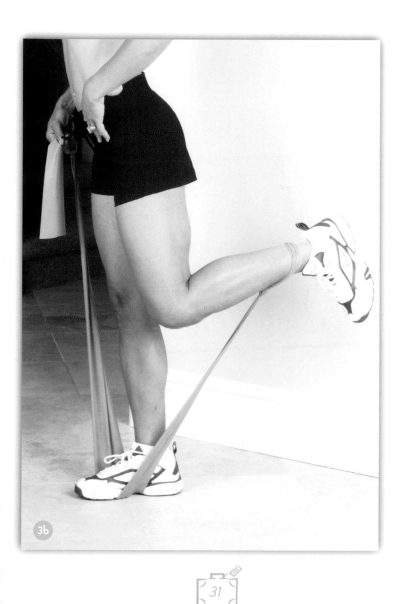

REAR LEG RAISES

Lift "leashed" foot to the rear, keeping the leg straight. The foot you are lifting should be externally rotated (4a). Only lift the leg as high as you can without feeling it in the lower back (4b). It may be quite a small movement, but it is very effective for the gluteus/buttocks.

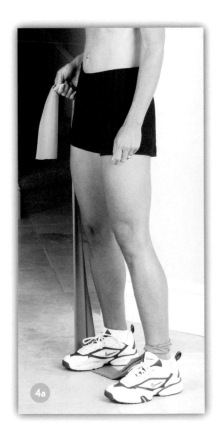

4a

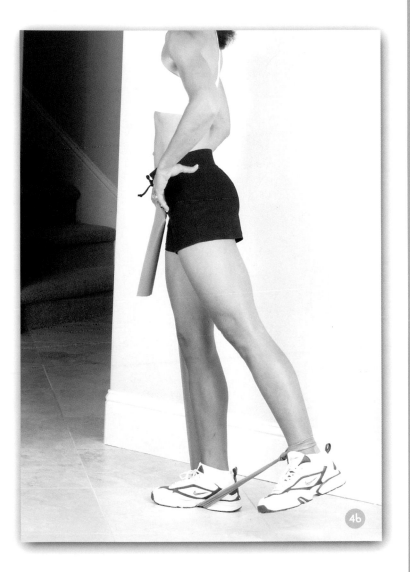

SQUATS

Stand on band, toes forward, feet just wider than shoulders. Depending on your desired resistance, hands should grip the band and remain at thighs, hips, or shoulders (5a). Bend knees to at least a 90° angle aiming the knees in the direction of the toes, "sitting back" while keeping your chest up and eyes forward (5b).

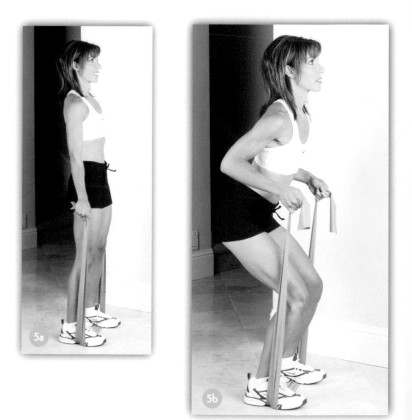

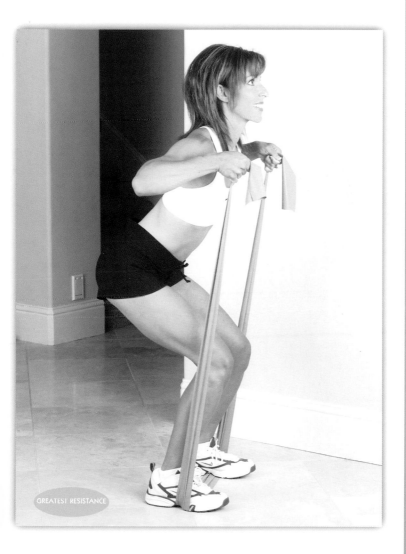

GREATEST RESISTANCE

OUTER THIGH/ADDUCTION

Standing on the band (6a), raise the leashed leg away from the body (6b). Return to starting position.

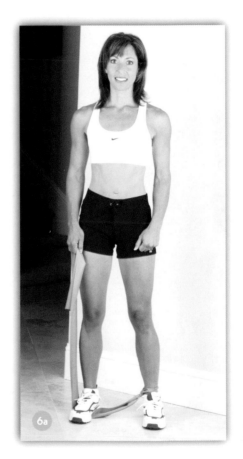

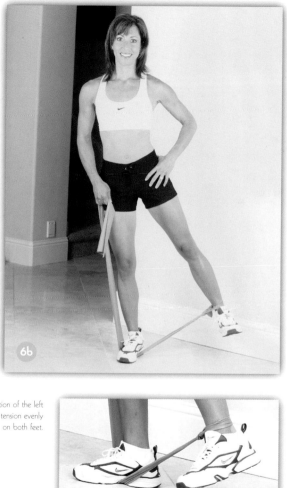

Notice the position of the left leg. Keep the tension evenly on both feet.

INNER THIGH/ABDUCTION

LEG RAISES

Lying on your side, prop yourself on the elbow directly under your shoulder. Have the leashed leg straightened in front of you with the rear knee bent. Place opposite foot on band to create tension (7a). Lift leashed leg and return to starting position (7b). Continue all repetitions on the leg, then switch legs.

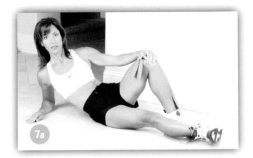

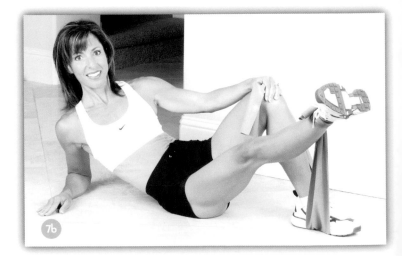

abdominals

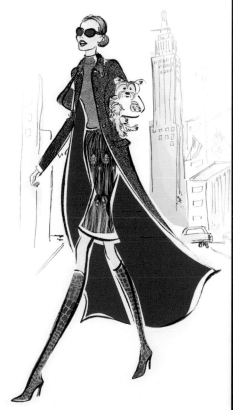

Yes, they are really there. Everyone has them. I am talking about your "six-pack." The way to tone and define your abdominal muscles, and to have a leaner torso, is by following a sound diet of lean proteins, a reasonable amount of carbohydrates and lots of veggies, and complete the following program three times a week. To reach the goal of a leaner torso, you should be completing 25 repetitions of each exercise.

The key thing to remember while doing this workout is to keep your neck and face relaxed. In addition, make sure your lower back is placed firmly on the floor. By maintaining this proper form, you will be isolating your stomach muscles to make sure all of your effort and hard work is targeted in the right area.

SIT-UPS/UPPER PRESS

Lie on your back with hands placed behind head, legs bent with feet on the floor (1a). Lift shoulders off of floor by moving into a forward position (1b). Return to initial position and repeat for all 25 repetitions.

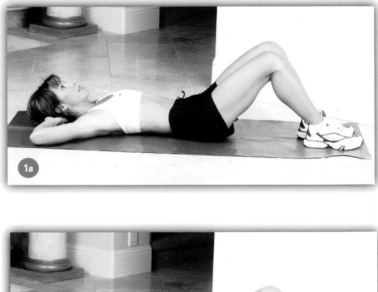

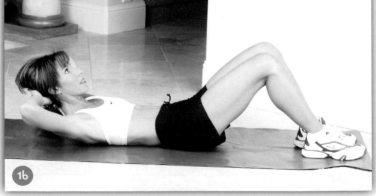

CRUNCH/LOWER PRESS

Lie on your back with hands placed behind head, legs bent with feet on the floor (2a). Lift tailbone off of floor, rolling hips up and back, pushing navel towards the floor (2b). Avoid swinging legs back and forth, this will engage other muscle groups and make the exercise less effective. It may be a very small range of motion. Return to initial position and repeat for all 25 repetitions.

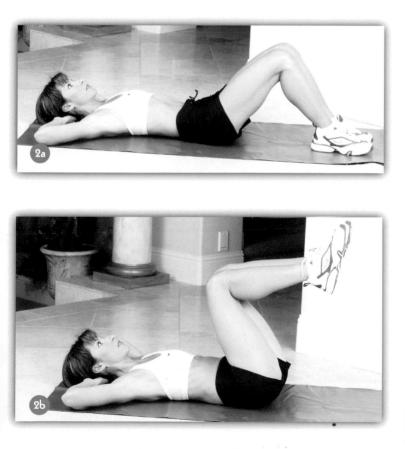

ABDOMINAL "BICYCLE"

Lie on your back with hands placed behind head. Bend and raise a leg 12 inches from floor. Press opposite shoulder toward raised leg's hip bone (3a). Internally rotate the trunk, visualizing the lowest rib moving toward the opposite hip bone. Alternate sides (3b) continually for 25 repetitions each.

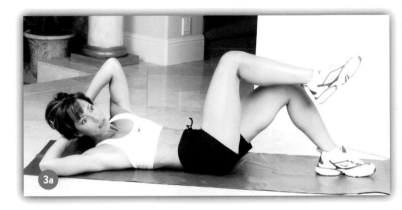

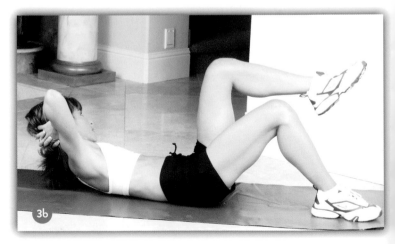

tracking your workouts

Taking notes is a great way to keep track of your workouts. Jot down the date of your routine, the time spent doing cardio warm-up, indicate which muscle group you exercised, how many repetitions, and how many sets you completed. This will help you remember your last session and challenge you to increase the intensity of your workout.

Date	Warm-up	Muscle Group	Reps	Sets	Comments

Date	Warm-up	Muscle Group	Reps	Sets	Comments

Date	Warm-up	Muscle Group	Reps	Sets	Comments

Date	Warm-up	Muscle Group	Reps	Sets	Comments

diet

tips

We hope you find these tips handy, not only for when you're traveling but, as a good rule of thumb for your eating habits in your day-to-day life.

- Choose fruits and sorbets for dessert options, or share a dessert.

- Select fat free salad dressings or ask for them to be served on the side.

- Size does matter; entrees are typically two to four times larger than a standard serving. Try to leave something on your plate.

- Go extra light on sauces even if it is a special request.

- Order a salad to start and have an appetizer as your main course.

- Have vegetables steamed without butter, order chicken and fish baked or grilled instead of fried, sautéed, or breaded.

- Eat only when you are hungry, regardless of the hour.

- Stop eating as soon as you feel satisfied, not when stuffed.

- Look for restaurants with lots of health-conscious options.

- Opt for berries or other fruit for dessert. Pair that with a flavored tea or a cappuccino to keep your hands busy.

- Stick with wine instead of sugar and fat-loaded mixed drinks.

- Drink water with meals to help your tummy feel fuller. Reach for water during the day instead of other sugar-laden drinks or snacks. See if that will satisfy you first.

- Try to select whole grain options with breads, and cereal products; they take longer for your body to digest and will keep your stomach satisfied for a longer period of time compared to their highly processed, white flour counterparts.

- Pack healthy snacks or protein bars from home to help you through any in-between meal snacking. This will help you avoid grabbing something that's not very nutritious from a vending machine or the hotel store.

- Keep a daily food diary. I know it sounds like work, but it helps to keep track of how much you're eating and also provides a way to remember restaurants you might want to visit on your next trip.

words of wisdom

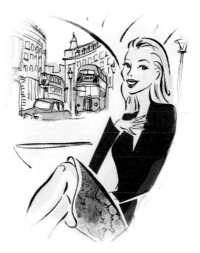

A true understanding of resistance training begins with an awareness of your body. Knowledge of basic anatomy will make your training so much more rewarding. Your body is not separate from you—it is not the enemy. It is the physical manifestation of you. So, when you look in the mirror, don't criticize your body. Instead, look at it with eyes that are filled with kindness, eyes that see you as you are today and define your attributes.

We hope these exercises will help you while you're on the road or at home. Our daily lives are full of very physical demands—including stress. It is vital that you manage these challenges with specific exercises to improve your strength, stamina, posture, and balance. Don't forget to work toward your goal of many happy, active years.

I know, I know. You don't workout at home, why would you workout when you're on the road? Think of this as a way to step out of your routine and into physical fitness. Take the time while you're traveling—for you. For the benefit of your mind and body. You might find that a workout is easy to fit into your schedule while you're on the road, and that now you can workout as a way of life at home too.

So when you're fed up with running, classes, weights and costly workout equipment, pick up this book. It is the only low-impact workout book that will go anywhere, help almost anyone, and really, truly works!

The Authors

Kari Eide—Kari has been a self-proclaimed "exercise junkie" for nearly 20 years. While attending California State University, Fresno, she took several courses in nutrition and physical education to further nurture her passion for physical fitness.

Lissa Mueller—Lissa has been active in the local fitness arena since opening Mueller Fitness with her husband, Vance in March of 1995. She is an A.C.E. Certified Personal Trainer and has developed fitness programs for clients of varying age and ability. She is an A.C.E. Certified Aerobic Instructor and Group Fitness Coordinator at Mueller Fitness in El Dorado Hills, CA. In addition, Lissa owns and operates her own Pilates studio and most recently added personal yoga instruction to her repertoire.

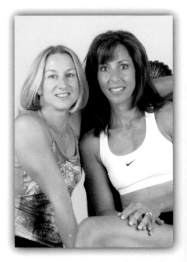

Lissa and Kari

Other fitness programs from
The Fitness Boutique

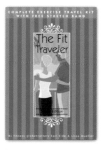

The Fit Traveler: Senior Edition
Specially created for the senior traveler over the age of 60. Over 23 of the most recommended exercises, fully illustrated with detailed instructions. Comes with light-resistance exercise band. Program was developed with a physical therapist, and a fitness expert.

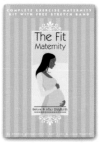

The Fit Maternity: Before & After Edition
Specially created for the expectant woman. Over 25 of the most recommended exercises, fully illustrated with detailed instructions. Comes with standard-resistance exercise band. Program was developed with an obstetrician and a fitness expert.

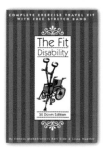

The Fit Disability: Sit-Down Workout
Specially created for the disabled person or injured, recovering patient. Over 21 of the most recommended exercises, fully illustrated with detailed instructions. Comes with light-resistance exercise band. Program was developed with a physical therapist, a chiropractor, and a fitness expert.

All fitness kits are available in bookstores, retailers, and travel concessionaires. Find a store at www.thefitnessboutique.com

Extra and replacement bands

Replacement bands may be purchased at retail stores,
spas, and boutiques, or by ordering online.

• Light-resistance bands •

• Medium-resistance bands (Standard-resistance) •

• Medium/heavy-resistance bands •

• Heavy-resistance bands •

• Extra heavy-resistance bands •

Videos and DVDs of *The Fit Traveler: Senior Edition* are available for presenting programs to groups of seniors.

Fitness trainers' pricing: If you lead fitness programs for groups of students, seniors, or disabled or recovery patients, please contact us for details on bulk discount purchases.

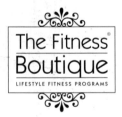

www.thefitnessboutique.com

The Fitenss Boutique, LLC.
P.O Box 5614
El Dorado Hills, CA 95762
1.800.963.0368

Published by
Publishers Design Group
1.800.587.6666
www.publishersdesign.com